ACXION FENTERMINA

WEIGHT LOSS

ULTIMATE GUIDE

Orion Tate

Copyright

© 2024 by Orion Tate

TABLE OF CONTENTS

Chapter 1: Introduction to Acxion Phentermine..... 7
What is Acxion Phentermine?.................7
How Does Acxion Phentermine Work?.................8
How Is Acxion Different from Other Forms of
Phentermine?.................10
Who Should Take Acxion Phentermine?.............11
Clinical Effectiveness of Acxion Phentermine....... 12
The Role of Acxion Phentermine in Weight Loss
Management.........................13
Chapter 2: Approved Uses and Benefits................. 6
Primary Use: Obesity and Weight Loss................. 6
Mechanism of Action in Weight Loss.................7
Secondary Benefits: Beyond Weight Loss............. 9
Weight Loss Expectations with Acxion Phentermine
12
Other Medical Considerations.............................14
Conclusion..................................... 15
**Chapter 3: Dosage and How to Take Acxion
Phentermine Safely.................................18**
Recommended Dosages of Acxion Phentermine. 18
Timing and Frequency of Administration..............19
Duration of Treatment................................. 21
Forms of Acxion Phentermine and Their Effects...22
How to Take Acxion Phentermine Safely............. 23
Warnings and Special Precautions...................... 26
Transitioning Off Acxion Phentermine.................29

Conclusion.. 29

**Chapter 4: Common Side Effects and Precautions..
20**

Common Side Effects of Acxion Phentermine...... 20

Severe Side Effects: When to Seek Immediate
Medical Attention...25

Drug Interactions and Contraindications............. 28

Long-Term Use and Dependence........................ 31

Who Should Avoid Acxion Phentermine?............ 32

Managing Side Effects....................................... 34

Conclusion... 35

**Chapter 5: Maximizing the Effectiveness of Acxion
Phentermine... 38**

Healthy Dietary Changes to Support Acxion
Phentermine...38

Exercise: Amplifying the Benefits of Acxion
Phentermine...42

The Importance of Hydration.............................45

The Role of Sleep in Weight Loss....................... 47

Behavioral Modifications and Psychological Support
48

Tracking Progress and Adjusting Strategies......... 50

Conclusion... 52

Chapter 6: Frequently Asked Questions (FAQ).....54

1. How Long Does It Take to See Results with
Acxion Phentermine?.. 54

2. What Happens When I Stop Taking Acxion
Phentermine?...55

3. Can I Drink Alcohol While Taking Acxion
Phentermine?...57

4. Will I Gain the Weight Back After Stopping Acxion Phentermine?...............58

5. How Much Weight Can I Expect to Lose with Acxion Phentermine?...............60

6. Can I Take Acxion Phentermine If I Have High Blood Pressure?...............61

7. Is Acxion Phentermine Safe for Long-Term Use?. 62

8. Can Acxion Phentermine Affect My Mood or Mental Health?...............63

9. Is Acxion Phentermine Addictive?...............64

10. Can Acxion Phentermine Be Taken Alongside Other Medications?...............65

Conclusion...............67

1. Behavioral Therapy and Counseling...............69

2. Nutritional Counseling and Meal Planning........72

3. Physical Therapy and Fitness Training...........74

4. Alternative Weight Loss Medications...............76

5. Surgical and Non-Surgical Weight Loss Procedures...............79

6. Mind-Body Practices and Stress Management. 82

Conclusion...............84

Chapter 8: Success Stories and Real-Life Results... 86

Success Story #1: Maria – 40 Pounds Lost in 12 Weeks...............87

Success Story #2: John – Overcoming a Plateau. 89

Success Story #3: Ana – Losing Weight with PCOS 92

Success Story #4: David – Losing Weight for Heart

Health...94

Lessons from Success Stories............................96

Conclusion... 98

1. Assessing Your Weight Loss Goals.............. 100

2. Are You Ready for Lifestyle Changes?.......... 102

3. Understanding the Risks and Benefits............ 104

4. Finding the Right Support System.................. 106

5. The Role of Medical Supervision................... 108

6. Moving Forward: Is Acxion Phentermine Right for You?.. 110

Conclusion: Sustaining Weight Loss Long-Term. 112

Final Thoughts...114

Chapter 1: Introduction to Acxion Phentermine

What is Acxion Phentermine?

Acxion Phentermine is a prescription medication primarily used for the short-term management of obesity. It is an anorectic or appetite suppressant, which means it helps reduce hunger sensations in individuals who are overweight or have obesity. The active ingredient in Acxion is **phentermine**, a stimulant that works on the central nervous system (CNS) to control appetite.

Phentermine has been widely used for weight loss since its approval by the U.S. Food and Drug Administration (FDA) in 1959. Acxion, in particular, is a brand commonly prescribed in countries like Mexico and is known for its specific formulation that delivers controlled doses of phentermine. It is generally prescribed to individuals with a **Body Mass Index (BMI) of 30 or higher**, or for those with a BMI of 27 or higher who also suffer from obesity-related conditions such as **hypertension, type 2 diabetes**, or **dyslipidemia**.

The primary goal of Acxion Phentermine is to assist individuals in losing weight through the suppression of appetite, which, when combined with a healthy diet and exercise regimen, can lead to significant reductions in body weight over a period of weeks to months.

How Does Acxion Phentermine Work?

Phentermine belongs to a class of drugs known as **sympathomimetic amines**. Its mechanism of action is similar to that of **amphetamine**-like medications. By stimulating the release of **norepinephrine** and other neurotransmitters in the brain, phentermine activates the "fight or flight" response. This leads to a decrease in hunger and an increase in energy expenditure.

More specifically, phentermine works by affecting the hypothalamus—the part of the brain that controls appetite. By promoting the release of norepinephrine, dopamine, and serotonin, it alters the communication between the nervous system and the brain, reducing the sensation of hunger. It also increases levels of energy, which can motivate individuals to engage in physical activity and, in turn, further enhance weight loss.

Though effective in suppressing appetite, Acxion Phentermine is typically prescribed for **short-term use** (up to 12 weeks), as the body can build up tolerance to the medication over time. It is not intended to be a long-term solution for weight loss but rather a **kick-start** to help individuals develop healthier habits that they can maintain after discontinuing the medication.

How Is Acxion Different from Other Forms of Phentermine?

Phentermine is available under various brand names, including **Adipex-P**, **Ionamin**, and generic versions. Acxion, however, is primarily marketed in Mexico and Latin America, and it is known for its specific formulation, which may come in different **dosages** and **delivery systems** compared to its U.S. counterparts. Common forms of Acxion include **immediate-release tablets** and **extended-release capsules**.

The most commonly prescribed forms of Acxion come in **15 mg** or **30 mg** doses, allowing doctors to adjust treatment according to the patient's needs. In some cases, extended-release versions are available, which release the medication over an extended period to provide prolonged appetite suppression throughout the day.

This flexibility in dosing and formulation allows for a more personalized approach to weight management, ensuring that each patient receives the appropriate level of medication to achieve optimal results.

Who Should Take Acxion Phentermine?

Acxion Phentermine is typically prescribed to individuals who are **medically obese**, meaning they have a **BMI** of 30 or higher, or a BMI of 27 or higher if they have weight-related health conditions such as **type 2 diabetes, high blood pressure**, or **high cholesterol**. Obesity is defined as a **chronic medical**

condition characterized by an excess of body fat, which increases the risk of numerous health issues, including cardiovascular disease, metabolic syndrome, and joint problems.

Patients who are eligible for Acxion Phentermine must be committed to a comprehensive weight-loss program that includes **dietary changes, increased physical activity**, and **behavioral therapy**. Phentermine alone is not a magic pill; its success relies heavily on the patient's ability to make and maintain healthier lifestyle choices.

Clinical Effectiveness of Acxion Phentermine

Numerous clinical trials have demonstrated that phentermine, including Acxion, is effective in promoting weight loss when used as part of a supervised weight-loss program. Patients can typically expect to lose approximately **5% to 10% of their**

initial body weight over the course of 12 weeks. This amount of weight loss has been shown to have meaningful health benefits, including improved **blood pressure, blood sugar levels**, and **cholesterol levels.**

Phentermine's effectiveness tends to decrease after the first few months of use, which is why it is recommended only for short-term therapy. Long-term success in weight management requires continued adherence to lifestyle changes after discontinuing the medication.

The Role of Acxion Phentermine in Weight Loss Management

In modern medical practice, obesity is often treated as a chronic, relapsing condition. The initial period of rapid weight loss achieved with the help of Acxion Phentermine serves to motivate patients and improve their health status enough to encourage continued efforts. However, **lifestyle modification** remains the cornerstone of sustainable weight loss. Acxion Phentermine is meant to serve as an **adjunct** to these modifications, not a substitute for them.

Additionally, Acxion Phentermine may be recommended for patients who have struggled to lose weight through conventional means alone. Many patients who are unable to control their weight through diet and exercise benefit from the appetite-suppressing effects of Acxion, which helps them break unhealthy eating patterns and adopt new habits.

In summary, Acxion Phentermine is a valuable tool for initiating weight loss in individuals with obesity or weight-related health problems. However, its use should always be part of a broader, long-term approach to weight management, emphasizing the importance of healthy eating, regular exercise, and behavioral changes to ensure lasting results.

Chapter 2: Approved Uses and Benefits

Primary Use: Obesity and Weight Loss

Acxion Phentermine is approved primarily for the **short-term treatment of obesity**. Obesity is defined by a **Body Mass Index (BMI)** of 30 or higher, or a BMI of 27 or higher in individuals with **weight-related comorbidities**, such as **hypertension (high blood pressure), type 2 diabetes**, or **dyslipidemia (abnormal cholesterol levels)**. Obesity is a complex and chronic condition that increases the risk of several serious health problems, including **heart disease, stroke, certain types of cancer**, and **joint disorders** like osteoarthritis.

Phentermine is typically prescribed for individuals who have **failed to lose weight through diet and exercise alone**. It is most effective when used as part of a comprehensive weight loss program that includes **caloric restriction, regular physical activity**, and, in some cases, **behavioral counseling**. The medication is designed to help patients **kick-start their weight loss efforts** by curbing appetite, making it easier to stick to a reduced-calorie diet.

In clinical practice, Acxion Phentermine is generally prescribed for short-term use, typically for **12 weeks**. It is important to note that phentermine is not a long-term solution for obesity management. Rather, it is intended to be used as an **adjunctive therapy** to facilitate the transition to a healthier lifestyle that will continue long after the medication is discontinued.

Mechanism of Action in Weight Loss

The primary way Acxion Phentermine promotes weight loss is by acting as an **anorectic**, meaning it suppresses appetite. By targeting neurotransmitters in the brain, phentermine affects the **hypothalamus**, a region that regulates hunger and satiety. Specifically, it increases the levels of **norepinephrine**, **dopamine**, and **serotonin** in the brain, creating a sensation of fullness, or **satiety**, that reduces the urge to eat.

Additionally, phentermine has mild **thermogenic properties**, meaning it can slightly increase the body's **basal metabolic rate** (BMR), which is the rate at which the body burns calories while at rest. This increase in metabolism, combined with the decreased appetite, helps promote a **caloric deficit**, which is essential for weight loss. When the body burns more calories than it consumes, it begins to use stored fat for energy, resulting in weight reduction.

While these effects are potent, phentermine is **not a cure for obesity**, nor is it a substitute for the necessary lifestyle changes. It is most effective when used in conjunction with **behavioral interventions**, including proper diet and exercise routines. These changes must be maintained beyond the period of medication use to ensure that the weight loss is sustainable.

Secondary Benefits: Beyond Weight Loss

In addition to its primary function of aiding in weight loss, Acxion Phentermine may offer several **secondary health benefits**. Because obesity is often linked to a range of metabolic disorders, reducing body weight can have a significant positive impact on overall health.

1. **Improvement in Cardiovascular Health**:

   By reducing body fat, particularly **visceral fat** (the fat stored around internal organs), weight loss can lead to improvements in **blood pressure, cholesterol levels,** and overall **heart health.** Studies have shown that even a **5-10% reduction in body weight** can result in lower blood pressure and decreased levels of **LDL ("bad") cholesterol** and **triglycerides,** while increasing **HDL ("good") cholesterol.** These changes help lower the risk of developing heart disease, the leading cause of death among individuals with obesity.

2. **Improved Glycemic Control in Type 2 Diabetes:** Weight loss has been shown to significantly improve **insulin sensitivity** and reduce **blood glucose levels** in individuals with **type 2 diabetes.** By losing weight, patients with diabetes may require lower doses of insulin or other diabetes medications, and in some cases, they

may even be able to achieve **remission** of their condition. Phentermine, by facilitating initial weight loss, may contribute to these metabolic improvements.

3. **Reduction in Obstructive Sleep Apnea**:

Obesity is a significant risk factor for **obstructive sleep apnea (OSA)**, a condition in which the airway becomes blocked during sleep, causing breathing interruptions. Weight loss can reduce the severity of OSA by decreasing fat deposits around the neck and upper airway, which in turn can improve **sleep quality** and reduce related risks such as **daytime fatigue**, **high blood pressure**, and **heart disease**.

4. **Enhanced Mobility and Joint Health**:

For individuals suffering from **osteoarthritis** or joint pain due to excess weight, even modest weight loss can relieve pressure on weight-bearing joints such as the knees, hips, and spine. Reduced strain on these joints can improve **mobility**, decrease **pain**, and enhance **quality of life**.

5. **Potential Psychological Benefits**:

Obesity is often associated with **mental health issues**, including **depression, anxiety**, and **low self-esteem**. While phentermine itself is not a treatment for these conditions, successful weight loss can lead to improved body image, increased confidence, and overall **emotional well-being**. For some individuals, losing weight may reduce the stigma they experience due to obesity, potentially improving social interactions and mental health.

Weight Loss Expectations with Acxion Phentermine

The amount of weight lost while taking Acxion Phentermine can vary depending on several factors, including the **individual's starting weight, adherence to lifestyle changes**, and **duration of treatment**. On average, clinical studies suggest that patients taking phentermine can expect to lose approximately **3-5% of their initial body weight** over a 12-week period. In some cases, more substantial weight loss of **5-10%** or more may be achieved, particularly when the medication is used in conjunction with a structured diet and exercise plan.

It is important for patients to have **realistic expectations** regarding their weight loss goals. Rapid weight loss is not always sustainable, and gradual, consistent progress is more likely to lead to **long-term success**. Moreover, the **amount of weight loss** needed to achieve meaningful health benefits is often less than what patients may initially expect. Research indicates that losing **just 5-10% of body weight** can result in significant improvements in **blood pressure, cholesterol levels,** and **blood sugar control,** even if the patient remains overweight according to BMI standards.

Other Medical Considerations

While Acxion Phentermine is highly effective for promoting short-term weight loss, its use must be carefully monitored due to potential **side effects** and **risks** (which will be discussed in greater detail in later chapters). It is essential that patients **consult their healthcare provider** regularly during treatment to ensure that the medication is working effectively and that any adverse effects are managed properly.

Furthermore, because phentermine is a **controlled substance** (classified as **Schedule IV** in the U.S.), it has a potential for **abuse or dependency**. Therefore, it is prescribed with caution, particularly for individuals with a history of substance use disorders or psychological conditions.

Patients are also encouraged to **transition off phentermine gradually**, under medical supervision, to avoid regaining weight after discontinuation. Maintaining lifestyle changes—such as a balanced diet and regular physical activity—is crucial for long-term success, as the body's metabolism may adjust once the medication is stopped, making weight maintenance more challenging.

Conclusion

In summary, Acxion Phentermine is a powerful tool in the treatment of obesity, particularly for individuals who have struggled to lose weight through conventional methods alone. By suppressing appetite and slightly boosting metabolism, it enables patients to make the initial progress needed to develop healthier eating and exercise habits. While the primary benefit of Acxion Phentermine is **weight loss**, secondary health improvements, such as enhanced **cardiovascular health**, better **glycemic control**, and improved **mobility**, are also important outcomes of successful treatment.

It is essential for individuals considering Acxion Phentermine to understand that the medication is **not a stand-alone solution**. Its effectiveness depends on a **comprehensive approach** that incorporates lifestyle changes, medical supervision, and behavioral support to ensure that weight loss is sustained over

time.

Chapter 3: Dosage and How to Take Acxion Phentermine Safely

Recommended Dosages of Acxion Phentermine

Acxion Phentermine is available in various **dosage forms** and **strengths** to suit the individual needs of each patient. The two most common forms are **immediate-release tablets** and **extended-release capsules**. The standard dosages typically prescribed are:

- **Acxion 15 mg** tablets: Immediate-release form, generally taken once or twice a day.

- **Acxion 30 mg** tablets: Immediate-release form, taken once daily, usually in the morning.

- **Acxion 30 mg** extended-release capsules: Taken once daily, providing a prolonged effect throughout the day.

The appropriate dosage depends on several factors, including the patient's **starting weight, medical history, response to treatment,** and **tolerance to the medication.** The initial dose is often lower (15 mg) to assess how the patient reacts to the medication. Based on the response and the presence of any side effects, the dose may be increased to 30 mg if deemed necessary by the healthcare provider.

Timing and Frequency of Administration

The timing of Acxion Phentermine administration is crucial to maximizing its effectiveness while minimizing potential side effects, particularly **insomnia.** Since phentermine has **stimulant-like properties,** it can interfere with sleep if taken too late in the day.

- **Immediate-release tablets** are generally taken **once daily**, in the morning, before or within **1 to 2 hours after breakfast**. For some patients, a **split dose** may be recommended, with the second dose taken in the early afternoon to maintain appetite suppression throughout the day.

- **Extended-release capsules** are typically taken **once in the morning**, as they release the medication gradually over several hours, providing more sustained appetite control throughout the day.

Patients should avoid taking Acxion Phentermine in the **late afternoon or evening**, as this can lead to difficulty falling asleep. **Missed doses** should not be doubled. If a dose is missed, it should be skipped, and the next dose should be taken at the regular time the following day to avoid overstimulation.

Duration of Treatment

Phentermine, including Acxion, is intended for **short-term use**. Most healthcare providers prescribe it for a duration of **12 weeks** or less. The body can develop a **tolerance** to the appetite-suppressing effects of phentermine over time, meaning the medication may become less effective after prolonged use.

The short-term nature of Acxion Phentermine is partly due to this **decreasing efficacy** and the potential for **side effects** or **dependency**. Phentermine is a **Schedule IV controlled substance**, meaning it has a potential for abuse or dependence, though this risk is considered lower than that of stronger stimulant medications like amphetamines.

In some cases, a healthcare provider may recommend **repeating the treatment** after a period of discontinuation if the patient has not achieved their weight loss goals. However, repeated courses of phentermine should only be considered under strict medical supervision.

Forms of Acxion Phentermine and Their Effects

Acxion Phentermine comes in **immediate-release** and **extended-release** forms. Understanding the differences between these two types is important for optimizing treatment:

- **Immediate-release tablets**: These tablets dissolve and release phentermine quickly into the bloodstream, providing a **rapid onset** of appetite suppression. They are best suited for patients who need **short bursts of control**, often around mealtimes.

- **Extended-release capsules**: These capsules are designed to release the medication slowly over time, ensuring a more **steady level of appetite suppression** throughout the day. This form is ideal for patients who struggle with hunger over extended periods and need more sustained control without the need for multiple daily doses.

Each form has its advantages, and the decision about which form to use should be made based on the patient's **lifestyle, eating patterns**, and **response to the medication**.

How to Take Acxion Phentermine Safely

Taking Acxion Phentermine safely involves **adhering to prescribed dosages** and **following specific instructions** to avoid potential side effects and complications. Below are key points for safe use:

1. **Take the Medication Exactly as Prescribed**:
   Always follow the dosing instructions provided by your

healthcare provider. Do not take more or less than the prescribed dose, and do not take the medication for longer than directed. Overuse of Acxion can lead to **serious side effects** or **dependency**.

2. **Take Acxion on an Empty Stomach**:

   Acxion Phentermine is most effective when taken before meals, typically before breakfast. This allows the medication to be absorbed quickly and start working to suppress appetite before your first meal of the day.

3. **Avoid Late-Afternoon or Evening Doses**:

   To reduce the risk of **insomnia**, avoid taking Acxion later in the day. If the medication interferes with sleep, consult your healthcare provider to discuss possible alternatives or dosage adjustments.

4. **Stay Hydrated**:

   Phentermine can cause **dry mouth**, which is a common side effect. Drink plenty of water throughout the day to stay hydrated and help alleviate this symptom. Additionally, staying hydrated can aid in overall weight loss and metabolic health.

5. **Do Not Combine with Other Weight Loss Medications**:

   Combining Acxion Phentermine with other **stimulant-based medications** or **appetite suppressants** can increase the risk of serious cardiovascular side effects, such as **elevated heart rate** and **high blood pressure**. Always consult your doctor before taking any additional medications or supplements.

6. **Regular Medical Checkups**:

Patients using Acxion Phentermine should have **regular checkups** to monitor their weight loss progress and assess for any potential side effects. Your healthcare provider may adjust your dose or recommend discontinuing the medication if any concerns arise.

7. **Follow a Healthy Diet and Exercise Plan**:

For Acxion Phentermine to be effective, it must be part of a comprehensive **weight loss plan** that includes dietary changes and regular physical activity. Relying on the medication alone without making these lifestyle changes may result in limited or temporary weight loss.

Warnings and Special Precautions

There are several precautions and warnings that patients must be aware of when using Acxion Phentermine to avoid complications:

- **Medical History**:

  Before starting Acxion Phentermine, it is important to inform your healthcare provider of your complete medical history, particularly if you have a history of **heart disease, hypertension, hyperthyroidism, glaucoma**, or **substance abuse**. These conditions may contraindicate the use of phentermine or require special monitoring during treatment.

- **Pregnancy and Breastfeeding**:

  Acxion Phentermine is classified as **Category X** in pregnancy, meaning it should not be used by pregnant women due to the risk of harm to the fetus. Similarly, the medication should not be used while breastfeeding, as it can pass into breast milk and potentially harm a nursing infant.

- **Mental Health Considerations**:

  Phentermine has been associated with **mood changes** in some individuals, including increased **anxiety** or **irritability**. Patients with a history of **depression** or **anxiety disorders** should use phentermine with caution and under close supervision by a healthcare provider.

- **Potential for Abuse or Dependency**:

  As a stimulant, phentermine has the potential for **abuse** or **psychological dependence**. Patients with a history of **substance use disorders** should be particularly cautious, and the medication should be used strictly as prescribed.

Transitioning Off Acxion Phentermine

When discontinuing Acxion Phentermine, it is essential to do so under medical supervision. Stopping the medication abruptly, especially after prolonged use, can lead to **withdrawal symptoms** such as **fatigue**, **depression**, and **increased appetite**.

Your healthcare provider may recommend **tapering off** the medication gradually to minimize these symptoms and to help you adjust to maintaining your weight without the appetite-suppressing effects of phentermine. Maintaining the **dietary** and **exercise** habits developed during treatment is critical to avoid regaining the weight lost during the medication period.

Conclusion

Acxion Phentermine is a powerful tool for short-term weight management when used according to prescribed dosages and under proper medical supervision. By following the appropriate guidelines, patients can maximize the benefits of the medication while minimizing the risk of side effects. The key to success with Acxion Phentermine lies not only in the medication itself but also in making lasting lifestyle changes that will ensure continued weight loss and improved health after the medication is discontinued.

As we continue, the next chapter will delve into the **common side effects** and **precautions** associated with Acxion Phentermine, helping readers understand how to recognize, manage, and avoid potential complications during treatment.

Chapter 4: Common Side Effects and Precautions

Common Side Effects of Acxion Phentermine

Like all medications, Acxion Phentermine can cause side effects, though not everyone will experience them. The most common side effects are usually mild and tend to diminish as the body adjusts to the medication. It is important to be aware of these potential side effects so that they can be managed effectively, and if necessary, addressed by a healthcare professional.

Here are some of the most frequently reported side effects associated with Acxion Phentermine:

1. **Dry Mouth (Xerostomia)**

   One of the most common side effects is **dry mouth**, which occurs as a result of reduced saliva production. This side effect can be uncomfortable but is generally manageable with increased **water intake**, the use of **sugar-free gum** or **lozenges**, and maintaining proper oral hygiene.

2. **Insomnia**

Due to its **stimulant properties**, Acxion Phentermine can interfere with sleep, causing **insomnia** or **difficulty falling asleep**. This effect is more likely if the medication is taken later in the day. To avoid sleep disturbances, Acxion should be taken in the morning or early afternoon. If insomnia persists, your doctor may adjust your dosage or recommend other strategies to improve sleep.

3. **Nervousness or Anxiety**

Some individuals may experience **nervousness, restlessness**, or **anxiety** as a result of the stimulating effects of phentermine. This can sometimes lead to a feeling of jitteriness or increased tension. Patients with pre-existing anxiety disorders may need to be monitored more closely or consider alternative treatments.

4. **Increased Heart Rate (Tachycardia)**

Acxion Phentermine can cause an increase in **heart rate**. This is a known effect of stimulant medications that impact the central nervous system. While mild increases in heart rate are generally not harmful, patients should monitor for signs of excessive heart palpitations or feelings of an irregular heartbeat (arrhythmia), and report these symptoms to their healthcare provider immediately.

5. **Elevated Blood Pressure**

Alongside tachycardia, Acxion Phentermine may lead to

elevated blood pressure in some individuals. Patients with a history of **hypertension** should use phentermine with caution, and regular blood pressure monitoring is recommended throughout the course of treatment. If blood pressure becomes too high, dosage adjustments or discontinuation of the medication may be necessary.

6. **Constipation**

Another side effect that some individuals may experience is **constipation**. This is typically due to decreased bowel motility, which can occur as a side effect of appetite suppression. To alleviate this issue, patients are encouraged to consume a diet high in **fiber**, drink plenty of water, and engage in regular physical activity.

7. **Headaches**

Headaches are another relatively common side effect

that may occur during the initial weeks of treatment as the body adjusts to the medication. In most cases, headaches are mild and can be managed with over-the-counter pain relievers, such as **ibuprofen** or **acetaminophen**.

8. **Dizziness**

Some patients report episodes of **dizziness** or **lightheadedness**, particularly during the early stages of treatment. It is important to avoid sudden movements, such as standing up too quickly, and to stay hydrated to reduce the likelihood of dizziness.

While these side effects are usually manageable, patients should always consult their healthcare provider if the symptoms persist or worsen.

Severe Side Effects: When to Seek Immediate Medical Attention

Although rare, Acxion Phentermine can cause more severe side effects that require immediate medical attention. Recognizing these symptoms early can help prevent serious health complications. Patients should contact their doctor or seek emergency medical care if they experience any of the following:

1. **Chest Pain or Shortness of Breath**

   Any sudden onset of **chest pain, tightness in the chest**, or **shortness of breath** should be treated as a medical emergency. These symptoms could indicate a serious cardiovascular event, such as a heart attack or pulmonary hypertension, both of which have been associated with the use of stimulant medications in some individuals.

2. **Severe Headache or Blurred Vision**

   A **severe headache** accompanied by **blurred vision** or **visual disturbances** may be a sign of dangerously elevated blood pressure, which requires immediate medical attention. This condition, known as **hypertensive crisis**, can lead to stroke or other life-threatening complications if left untreated.

3. **Severe Mood Changes**

   Although less common, some patients may experience **severe mood swings**, **agitation**, or **depression** while taking Acxion Phentermine. If these symptoms are accompanied by thoughts of self-harm or suicidal ideation, it is crucial to seek immediate psychological support.

4. **Irregular Heartbeat (Arrhythmia)**

While mild increases in heart rate are expected, an **irregular heartbeat** or **arrhythmia** can be dangerous. If you notice **fluttering, palpitations,** or an abnormally fast or slow heart rate, you should stop taking the medication and contact your doctor right away.

5. **Allergic Reactions**

Though rare, some individuals may have an allergic reaction to Acxion Phentermine. Symptoms of an allergic reaction include **hives, swelling of the face, lips, tongue,** or **throat,** and **difficulty breathing.** This is a medical emergency and requires immediate attention.

Drug Interactions and Contraindications

When taking Acxion Phentermine, it is essential to be aware of **potential drug interactions** that may increase the risk of side effects or reduce the effectiveness of the treatment. Certain medications and medical conditions are contraindicated with phentermine use.

- **Monoamine Oxidase Inhibitors (MAOIs):** Patients should not take Acxion Phentermine if they are currently using or have recently discontinued (within the last 14 days) **MAOI antidepressants.** The combination of MAOIs and phentermine can cause **hypertensive crisis**, a sudden and dangerous increase in blood pressure.

- **Other Stimulants**:

  Combining Acxion Phentermine with other stimulant medications, such as those used to treat **attention deficit hyperactivity disorder (ADHD)** (e.g., **amphetamine** or **methylphenidate**), can exacerbate side effects like **tachycardia** and **elevated blood pressure**. This combination should be avoided unless specifically directed by a healthcare provider.

- **Selective Serotonin Reuptake Inhibitors (SSRIs)**:

  Phentermine, including Acxion, may interact with **SSRIs**, which are commonly prescribed for depression and anxiety. This combination can increase the risk of a rare but serious condition known as **serotonin syndrome**, characterized by symptoms such as confusion, **agitation**, **rapid heart rate**, and **muscle rigidity**.

- **Heart Disease and Hypertension**:

  Acxion Phentermine should not be used by individuals with **severe heart disease**, **uncontrolled hypertension**, or a history of **stroke**. These conditions increase the risk of serious cardiovascular events, and the stimulant effects of phentermine can exacerbate these risks.

- **Hyperthyroidism and Glaucoma**:

  Patients with **hyperthyroidism** (overactive thyroid) or **glaucoma** should avoid using Acxion Phentermine, as it may worsen these conditions. Phentermine can increase intraocular pressure in glaucoma patients, potentially leading to further eye damage.

Long-Term Use and Dependence

Acxion Phentermine is classified as a **Schedule IV controlled substance**, indicating that it has a potential for **abuse** or **dependency**, though this risk is relatively low when used as prescribed. Long-term use of phentermine is not recommended due to the risk of developing **tolerance**. As tolerance builds, the appetite-suppressing effects of the medication may diminish, leading some patients to increase the dose without medical supervision, which can result in dangerous side effects.

Patients with a history of **substance use disorders** should be particularly cautious when using Acxion Phentermine, as they may be more vulnerable to developing psychological dependence on the drug. Healthcare providers typically prescribe phentermine for **short-term use only** (up to 12 weeks), and any extension of treatment should be carefully monitored.

Who Should Avoid Acxion Phentermine?

There are specific populations for whom Acxion Phentermine is not recommended due to the increased risk of adverse effects:

1. **Pregnant or Breastfeeding Women**

   Acxion Phentermine is contraindicated during **pregnancy** and **breastfeeding**. The medication is classified as **Category X**, meaning that it can cause harm to the fetus and should not be used during pregnancy. Similarly, the drug can be passed to an infant through breast milk, potentially causing harm.

2. **Individuals with a History of Cardiovascular Disease**

Patients with a history of **heart disease**, including **arrhythmias, coronary artery disease, congestive heart failure,** or a previous **heart attack,** should avoid phentermine due to the increased risk of serious cardiovascular side effects.

3. **Patients with Severe Uncontrolled Hypertension**

Acxion Phentermine can exacerbate **high blood pressure** and should not be used in individuals with **uncontrolled hypertension.** These patients should explore alternative weight loss options under the guidance of their healthcare provider.

4. **People with Psychological Disorders**

Individuals with a history of **severe mood disorders,** such as **schizophrenia** or **bipolar disorder,** should avoid using Acxion Phentermine. The stimulant effects of the medication can sometimes worsen mood swings, agitation, or delusions.

Managing Side Effects

For those experiencing mild side effects, several strategies can help reduce discomfort and improve overall tolerability:

- **Hydration and Oral Care:**

  Drinking plenty of water throughout the day can alleviate dry mouth, while maintaining proper oral hygiene can prevent any related dental issues.

- **Adequate Sleep Hygiene:**

  To manage insomnia, ensure you take the medication early in the day and establish a consistent sleep routine. Avoid caffeine and other stimulants in the evening.

- **Dietary Adjustments**:

  Eating a fiber-rich diet and staying hydrated can help alleviate constipation. Additionally, limiting **sodium intake** can help prevent elevated blood pressure.

- **Exercise and Stress Management**:

  Regular physical activity can not only boost weight loss but also improve mood, reduce anxiety, and help regulate sleep patterns. Practicing stress-relief techniques such as **meditation, yoga**, or **deep breathing exercises** can further help manage any stimulant-related restlessness.

Conclusion

Understanding the potential side effects and precautions associated with Acxion Phentermine is crucial for safe and effective use. While the medication can be a powerful tool for weight loss, it comes with risks that must be carefully managed. Patients should be fully informed about these risks and work closely with their healthcare provider to monitor their progress and make any necessary adjustments to their treatment plan.

In the next chapter, we will discuss strategies for **maximizing the effectiveness of Acxion Phentermine**, including complementary lifestyle changes that can enhance weight loss and ensure long-term success.

Chapter 5: Maximizing the Effectiveness of Acxion Phentermine

Acxion Phentermine is a powerful tool for weight loss, but its true effectiveness is maximized when it is used as part of a comprehensive lifestyle change. This chapter explores key strategies that can help patients achieve the best possible results while minimizing potential setbacks. The primary areas of focus include **diet, exercise, hydration, sleep,** and **behavioral modifications**. Together, these elements work in synergy with the medication to optimize weight loss and ensure long-term success.

Healthy Dietary Changes to Support Acxion Phentermine

A proper diet is the cornerstone of any successful weight loss plan. While Acxion Phentermine helps suppress appetite, making it easier to consume fewer calories, patients must focus on the **quality** of the foods they eat to achieve the best results. Below are dietary strategies that can enhance the effectiveness of Acxion:

1. **Caloric Deficit**

   The fundamental principle behind weight loss is creating a **caloric deficit**, which means consuming fewer calories than the body burns in a day. While Acxion helps reduce caloric intake by curbing appetite, patients should aim to eat **nutrient-dense, low-calorie foods** that provide essential vitamins and minerals without excessive calories. The caloric intake should be adjusted based on individual needs, but a general guideline for weight loss is to reduce daily caloric intake by **500 to 1,000 calories** from the baseline, which can result in a weight loss of **1 to 2 pounds per week.**

2. **Prioritize Protein-Rich Foods**

Protein is an essential macronutrient for weight loss because it helps preserve **lean muscle mass** while promoting **fat loss.** It also increases **satiety,** meaning patients feel fuller for longer periods, reducing the likelihood of overeating. Foods such as **lean meats, poultry, fish, eggs, beans,** and **low-fat dairy** products are excellent sources of protein that can be incorporated into daily meals.

3. **Low-Glycemic Index (GI) Carbohydrates**

To stabilize blood sugar levels and prevent energy crashes, patients should focus on consuming **low-GI carbohydrates,** which are digested slowly and provide a steady release of energy. Examples include **whole grains, oats, quinoa, sweet potatoes,** and **legumes**. These foods help maintain satiety and prevent the **blood sugar spikes** that can lead to cravings.

4. **Healthy Fats**

   Although fats are higher in calories than proteins and carbohydrates, **healthy fats** are essential for optimal health and can actually aid in weight loss when consumed in moderation. Sources of healthy fats include **avocados, nuts, seeds, olive oil,** and **fatty fish** like **salmon** and **tuna**. These fats can promote satiety and reduce the desire for processed snacks high in unhealthy fats.

5. **Avoid Processed Foods and Sugary Drinks**

   Highly processed foods and sugary beverages, such as

sodas, packaged snacks, and fast food, are typically high in **empty calories** and offer little nutritional value. These foods can spike blood sugar levels and lead to increased hunger soon after eating. Instead, focus on **whole foods** that are minimally processed and rich in nutrients.

6. **Smaller, More Frequent Meals**

Eating **smaller, more frequent meals** throughout the day can help prevent overeating at any single meal. This approach can keep energy levels stable and support weight loss efforts by maintaining a **steady metabolic rate**. It is especially helpful for those who may still experience hunger despite taking Acxion.

Exercise: Amplifying the Benefits of Acxion Phentermine

Exercise is a critical component of any weight loss program. While Acxion Phentermine helps reduce caloric intake, exercise boosts the number of calories burned and supports long-term weight maintenance. A balanced exercise routine should include both **cardiovascular exercise** and **strength training** to maximize fat loss and improve overall fitness.

1. **Cardiovascular Exercise (Cardio)**

   Cardio activities such as **walking, running, cycling, swimming,** and **aerobic classes** increase the heart rate and promote calorie burning. Patients are encouraged to aim for **150 minutes of moderate-intensity cardio** or **75 minutes of vigorous-intensity cardio** per week, as recommended by most health guidelines. Starting with low-impact activities like walking can be effective for beginners and gradually building intensity can yield better results over time.

2. **Strength Training**

Building **lean muscle mass** through strength training is essential for weight loss because muscle tissue burns more calories at rest than fat tissue. Strength training exercises, such as **weightlifting, bodyweight exercises** (e.g., squats, lunges, push-ups), and **resistance band exercises**, should be performed **2 to 3 times per week**. These exercises not only help tone and shape the body but also enhance **metabolic efficiency**, leading to greater calorie expenditure even when at rest.

3. **Incorporating Movement Throughout the Day**

Beyond structured exercise sessions, it is important to increase overall daily movement. Activities such as taking the stairs instead of the elevator, walking during breaks, and standing rather than sitting for long periods can contribute to additional calorie burn. These small changes can make a significant difference over time.

4. **Finding Enjoyable Activities**

One of the keys to maintaining a long-term exercise routine is finding activities that are enjoyable. Whether it's **dancing, hiking, swimming,** or **playing a sport,** incorporating activities that bring joy can help ensure consistency and reduce the likelihood of abandoning the exercise plan.

The Importance of Hydration

Staying hydrated is essential for overall health and can also aid in weight loss. Acxion Phentermine can cause **dry mouth**, which can lead to discomfort if not properly managed. Drinking sufficient water can help alleviate this side effect while also promoting fat metabolism and digestion.

- **Water Intake Guidelines**:

  The general recommendation for water intake is to drink **8 glasses of water per day** (about 2 liters), but individual needs can vary depending on factors like activity level, climate, and body size. Some experts suggest drinking **half your body weight in ounces** as a good guideline (for example, a 160-pound person would aim for 80 ounces of water per day).

- **Water as a Weight Loss Aid**:

  Drinking water before meals can help reduce overall

calorie intake by promoting **early satiety**. Additionally, sometimes **thirst** is mistaken for hunger, so staying hydrated can help prevent unnecessary snacking.

The Role of Sleep in Weight Loss

Sleep plays a critical role in weight management. Lack of sleep can disrupt hormones involved in hunger and satiety, leading to **increased appetite** and **cravings for unhealthy foods**. Studies have shown that sleep deprivation increases levels of **ghrelin** (the hunger hormone) and decreases levels of **leptin** (the hormone that signals fullness), which can sabotage weight loss efforts.

- **Aim for 7-9 Hours of Sleep per Night**:
  To support weight loss and overall health, adults should aim for **7 to 9 hours of sleep** each night. Patients taking

Acxion Phentermine should be mindful of the medication's **stimulant effects**, which can interfere with sleep if taken too late in the day. Establishing a regular **sleep routine** and creating a **calm, relaxing sleep environment** can help improve sleep quality.

- **Tips for Better Sleep:**

    o Avoid caffeine and other stimulants in the late afternoon and evening.

    o Establish a consistent bedtime and wake-up time, even on weekends.

    o Create a relaxing bedtime routine, such as reading or taking a warm bath.

    o Ensure the bedroom is cool, dark, and quiet to promote restful sleep.

Behavioral Modifications and Psychological Support

Achieving lasting weight loss often requires more than just physical changes; **behavioral modifications** and **psychological support** are key components of a comprehensive weight loss plan. Acxion Phentermine can help control hunger, but it is important to address the underlying habits and emotions that contribute to overeating.

1. **Behavioral Therapy**

   Cognitive-behavioral therapy (CBT) can be highly effective for individuals struggling with **emotional eating, binge eating**, or difficulty maintaining dietary changes. CBT helps patients identify and change negative thought patterns and behaviors that lead to overeating. It also provides practical tools for managing stress, setting realistic goals, and developing **healthy coping mechanisms**.

2. Mindful Eating

Practicing **mindful eating** can help patients develop a healthier relationship with food. This involves paying close attention to hunger and fullness cues, eating slowly, and savoring each bite. Mindful eating can prevent **overeating** and promote a more enjoyable eating experience.

3. Support Groups and Counseling

For many individuals, **emotional support** is crucial during the weight loss journey. **Support groups**, either online or in person, can provide encouragement and accountability. Talking to a counselor or therapist can also help address any **psychological barriers** to weight loss, such as low self-esteem, anxiety, or past trauma.

Tracking Progress and Adjusting Strategies

Monitoring progress is an important aspect of staying motivated and adjusting the weight loss plan as needed. Regularly tracking **weight, body measurements, physical activity**, and **food intake** can provide valuable insights into what is working and where adjustments may be necessary.

1. **Keep a Food Journal**

   A **food journal** can help patients stay accountable and mindful of what they are eating. It can also help identify any patterns or triggers that lead to overeating. Tracking food intake can also help ensure that patients are meeting their nutritional needs while maintaining a caloric deficit.

2. **Monitor Physical Activity**

   Using fitness trackers or apps to monitor **daily steps** and **exercise** can provide motivation to stay active and achieve fitness goals. Setting realistic, measurable goals and celebrating progress can boost confidence and help maintain consistency.

3. **Regular Weigh-Ins**

Weighing in once a week can help track progress without causing unnecessary stress or discouragement. Since weight can fluctuate due to factors like water retention or muscle gain, it is important to focus on overall trends rather than daily fluctuations.

Conclusion

Maximizing the effectiveness of Acxion Phentermine requires more than just taking the medication as prescribed. By adopting a **balanced diet**, engaging in **regular physical activity**, staying **hydrated**, getting sufficient **sleep**, and making key **behavioral** changes, patients can significantly enhance their weight loss results and improve their overall health. These lifestyle changes not only support the medication's effects but also provide a foundation for **sustainable weight management** after the treatment period ends.

In the next chapter, we will address **Frequently Asked Questions (FAQ)** about Acxion Phentermine, offering additional guidance and clarity on common concerns that patients may have during their weight loss journey.

Chapter 6: Frequently Asked Questions (FAQ)

A comprehensive understanding of **Acxion Phentermine** requires addressing common questions that patients often have regarding the medication. This section is designed to clarify doubts, provide practical advice, and ensure safe and effective use of Acxion Phentermine.

---

1. How Long Does It Take to See Results with Acxion Phentermine?

The results of Acxion Phentermine can vary from person to person, depending on factors such as starting weight, adherence to diet and exercise, and overall health. However, most patients begin to notice **appetite suppression** within a few days of starting the medication.

On average, significant weight loss typically begins to be noticeable after **2 to 4 weeks** of treatment. Studies suggest that patients may lose approximately **5% of their initial body weight** over the course of **12 weeks** when using Acxion Phentermine alongside a reduced-calorie diet and regular physical activity.

It is important to remember that weight loss should be gradual and consistent. Rapid weight loss can lead to muscle loss, nutrient deficiencies, and other health issues. A safe and sustainable weight loss goal is typically **1 to 2 pounds per week**.

---

2. What Happens When I Stop Taking Acxion Phentermine?

After discontinuing Acxion Phentermine, patients may experience an increase in appetite as the appetite-suppressing effects of the medication wear off. To prevent **regaining the weight** that was lost, it is essential to have developed healthy eating and exercise habits during the treatment period.

Some strategies to maintain weight loss after stopping Acxion Phentermine include:

- **Continuing a balanced diet** with appropriate portion control.

- **Staying physically active** by engaging in regular exercise.

- **Monitoring weight regularly** to detect and address any early signs of weight regain.

- Seeking **behavioral support** if necessary, such as counseling or joining a weight loss support group.

Patients should transition off the medication gradually, under the supervision of their healthcare provider, to avoid abrupt changes that could lead to weight gain or other side effects.

---

3. Can I Drink Alcohol While Taking Acxion Phentermine?

It is generally not recommended to consume **alcohol** while taking Acxion Phentermine. Both alcohol and phentermine can have stimulant effects on the central nervous system, and combining the two can increase the risk of side effects, such as:

- **Increased heart rate and blood pressure**.

- **Dizziness or lightheadedness.**

- **Mood changes** or **anxiety.**

- **Impaired judgment or coordination**, which could increase the risk of accidents or injury.

Additionally, alcohol contains **empty calories**, which can hinder weight loss efforts. If you choose to drink alcohol while on Acxion Phentermine, it is important to do so in moderation and be aware of how your body responds.

---

4. Will I Gain the Weight Back After Stopping Acxion Phentermine?

Weight regain is a common concern after discontinuing Acxion Phentermine. The key to preventing this is to maintain the

lifestyle changes that were developed during treatment, such as a healthy diet, regular exercise, and portion control.

Phentermine is intended to be a **short-term aid** to help establish these habits, not a long-term solution for weight management. Patients who rely solely on the medication without making sustainable lifestyle changes are more likely to experience weight regain.

To minimize the risk of gaining weight after stopping Acxion Phentermine, it is important to:

- Continue **monitoring food intake** and **staying active**.
- Address any **emotional or psychological factors** that may contribute to overeating.
- Consider working with a **nutritionist** or **behavioral therapist** for ongoing support.

5. How Much Weight Can I Expect to Lose with Acxion Phentermine?

The amount of weight loss experienced while taking Acxion Phentermine varies by individual, but on average, patients can expect to lose **3-5% of their initial body weight** within the first **12 weeks** of treatment. This equates to approximately **5 to 10 pounds** for someone who weighs 200 pounds at the start of treatment.

The total weight loss will depend on several factors, including adherence to a **reduced-calorie diet**, the level of **physical activity**, and how the body responds to the medication. It is important to set **realistic goals** and focus on gradual, sustainable weight loss.

6. Can I Take Acxion Phentermine If I Have High Blood Pressure?

Patients with **controlled high blood pressure** (hypertension) may be able to take Acxion Phentermine, but they should do so under the close supervision of a healthcare provider. Phentermine can raise **heart rate** and **blood pressure**, so it is crucial to monitor these vital signs regularly during treatment.

For individuals with **uncontrolled hypertension**, Acxion Phentermine may not be recommended due to the risk of exacerbating cardiovascular issues. Always consult your doctor to assess whether it is safe for you to use phentermine if you have a history of high blood pressure or other cardiovascular conditions.

7. Is Acxion Phentermine Safe for Long-Term Use?

Acxion Phentermine is approved for **short-term use**, typically **up to 12 weeks**. It is not recommended for long-term use due to the risk of **tolerance**, **dependency**, and potential cardiovascular side effects. Over time, the body can develop a tolerance to the medication, meaning its appetite-suppressing effects may diminish, and higher doses would be required to achieve the same results.

For long-term weight management, patients should focus on **lifestyle changes**, including a healthy diet, exercise, and behavioral modifications. In some cases, healthcare providers may consider repeating a course of Acxion Phentermine after a period of discontinuation, but this should only be done under medical supervision.

---

8. Can Acxion Phentermine Affect My Mood or Mental Health?

Phentermine, including Acxion, is a **stimulant** that can affect the central nervous system, which means it may impact mood and mental health in some individuals. Potential mood-related side effects include:

- **Anxiety** or **nervousness.**

- **Irritability** or **restlessness.**

- **Mood swings** or **depression** (in rare cases).

Patients with a history of **mental health conditions**, such as

anxiety disorders, bipolar disorder, or **depression**, should

use Acxion Phentermine with caution and under close medical

supervision. If mood changes or mental health concerns arise

during treatment, it is important to consult with a healthcare

provider to determine the best course of action.

---

9. Is Acxion Phentermine Addictive?

Acxion Phentermine is classified as a **Schedule IV controlled**

substance, which means it has a potential for **abuse** and

dependence, although this risk is considered lower than with

stronger stimulants, such as amphetamines.

When used as prescribed and for short-term use, the risk of

addiction is low. However, individuals with a history of

substance use disorders should use Acxion with caution, as they may be at a higher risk for developing dependency on the medication.

If you are concerned about the possibility of addiction or dependency, discuss these concerns with your healthcare provider before starting treatment.

---

10. Can Acxion Phentermine Be Taken Alongside Other Medications?

Acxion Phentermine can interact with certain medications, so it is important to inform your healthcare provider of all medications you are currently taking, including **prescription drugs**, **over-the-counter medications**, and **herbal supplements**. Some notable interactions include:

- **Monoamine oxidase inhibitors (MAOIs)**: These medications, used to treat depression, should not be taken with phentermine due to the risk of a dangerous increase in blood pressure.

- **Other stimulants**: Combining phentermine with other stimulant medications (e.g., for ADHD) can increase the risk of cardiovascular side effects, such as elevated heart rate and blood pressure.

- **Selective serotonin reuptake inhibitors (SSRIs)**: Combining phentermine with SSRIs, commonly prescribed for depression or anxiety, can increase the risk of **serotonin syndrome**, a rare but serious condition.

Always consult with your healthcare provider to ensure that taking Acxion Phentermine alongside your other medications is safe.

Conclusion

This FAQ section addresses many of the common concerns and questions that arise when using Acxion Phentermine. Understanding the risks, benefits, and practical considerations surrounding this medication can help patients make informed decisions and use it effectively as part of their weight loss journey.

In the next chapter, we will explore **complementary therapies** and **alternative treatments** that can be used alongside Acxion Phentermine to enhance weight loss results and improve overall well-being.

Chapter 7: Complementary Therapies and Alternative Treatments

Acxion Phentermine can be highly effective in supporting weight loss when combined with lifestyle changes, but there are additional therapies and treatments that can further enhance its effectiveness. These complementary and alternative approaches focus on **behavioral changes, therapeutic interventions,** and **non-pharmacological treatments** that can help patients achieve long-term success in their weight loss journey.

In this chapter, we will explore several approaches, including **behavioral therapy, nutritional counseling, alternative weight loss medications,** and **non-surgical procedures.** Additionally, we will discuss how integrating **mental health support** and **physical therapy** can improve overall well-being.

1. Behavioral Therapy and Counseling

Behavioral therapy is an evidence-based approach that focuses on modifying unhealthy behaviors and habits that contribute to weight gain. The goal of behavioral therapy is to help patients develop long-lasting, sustainable lifestyle changes that can support their weight loss efforts long after they have stopped taking Acxion Phentermine.

Key components of behavioral therapy include:

- **Cognitive-Behavioral Therapy (CBT):**
  CBT is one of the most effective forms of therapy for managing weight-related behaviors. It helps individuals identify and change **negative thought patterns** and **emotional triggers** that lead to overeating. For example,

many people struggle with **emotional eating**, using food as a way to cope with stress, anxiety, or boredom. CBT helps patients replace these behaviors with healthier coping mechanisms, such as **exercise, mindfulness, or hobbies.**

- **Goal Setting and Self-Monitoring:**

Behavioral therapy often involves setting **specific, measurable, and achievable goals** related to diet and exercise. Patients are encouraged to track their progress through **food diaries, exercise logs**, and **regular weigh-ins**. This process of self-monitoring not only provides accountability but also helps individuals recognize patterns that may be hindering their weight loss progress.

- **Motivational Interviewing**:

  A key aspect of behavioral therapy is **motivational interviewing**, a counseling technique designed to help individuals overcome ambivalence about making lifestyle changes. It focuses on building internal motivation and self-efficacy, encouraging patients to take ownership of their health and weight loss journey.

For many individuals, combining Acxion Phentermine with behavioral therapy can be a powerful strategy for addressing both the **psychological** and **physical** aspects of weight management. Many healthcare providers recommend working with a **licensed therapist** or a **psychologist** specializing in weight loss to ensure comprehensive care.

2. Nutritional Counseling and Meal Planning

While Acxion Phentermine helps control appetite, long-term success in weight loss requires making **sustainable dietary changes**. **Nutritional counseling** is a valuable tool for individuals who need guidance on creating a balanced, nutrient-dense diet that supports weight loss while providing essential vitamins and minerals.

A **registered dietitian** or **nutritionist** can work with patients to:

- **Create Personalized Meal Plans**:

  Every individual has unique nutritional needs, and working with a professional can help patients design meal plans tailored to their specific goals, preferences, and lifestyle. Meal plans often focus on incorporating

whole foods, lean proteins, healthy fats, and **complex carbohydrates** to ensure a well-rounded diet.

- **Identify Nutritional Deficiencies:**

  Some individuals may struggle with nutrient deficiencies that can hinder weight loss or overall health. For example, deficiencies in **vitamin D, magnesium,** or **iron** can lead to **fatigue, slowed metabolism,** and **food cravings.** A nutritionist can identify these deficiencies and recommend dietary changes or supplements to correct them.

- **Portion Control and Mindful Eating:**

  Nutritional counseling can also help patients develop **portion control** strategies, which are essential for maintaining a caloric deficit without feeling deprived. **Mindful eating** techniques, such as **eating slowly** and

paying attention to hunger cues, can also help patients avoid overeating and make more conscious food choices.

Incorporating **regular check-ins** with a nutritionist can provide ongoing support, helping patients adjust their meal plans as they progress in their weight loss journey.

---

3. Physical Therapy and Fitness Training

For individuals who may have **limited mobility** or **chronic pain** due to obesity, working with a **physical therapist** can be an essential part of their weight loss program. Physical therapy helps patients develop safe and effective exercise routines that improve mobility, reduce pain, and increase overall fitness levels.

Benefits of physical therapy include:

- **Improved Joint Function**:

  Obesity can place excess strain on weight-bearing joints like the **knees, hips,** and **lower back,** leading to pain and discomfort during physical activity. A physical therapist can provide **targeted exercises** to strengthen muscles around the joints, improve flexibility, and reduce pain.

- **Posture and Balance**:

  Many individuals with obesity experience **poor posture** and **balance issues** due to the additional weight. Physical therapy can help improve **core strength** and **stability**, reducing the risk of falls and improving overall mobility.

- **Personalized Exercise Plans**:

  For individuals new to exercise or those with health limitations, physical therapists can design **low-impact exercise programs** that are safe and appropriate for their fitness level. These exercises may include activities like **water aerobics**, **walking**, or **cycling**, which are easier on the joints while still promoting weight loss.

For individuals who are more active or want to intensify their workouts, working with a **personal trainer** can be beneficial. A trainer can help set realistic fitness goals, develop **strength training routines**, and provide **motivation** and **accountability**.

---

4. Alternative Weight Loss Medications

In some cases, patients may not respond as expected to Acxion Phentermine or may experience side effects that make continued use difficult. There are several **alternative weight loss medications** approved by the FDA that can be considered, either as standalone treatments or in combination with other therapies.

Some of the commonly prescribed alternative medications include:

- **Orlistat (Xenical):**

  Orlistat works by inhibiting the absorption of dietary fat in the intestines, reducing overall caloric intake. It is available over-the-counter in a lower dose as **Alli** and as a prescription in higher doses. Orlistat is particularly helpful for individuals who have difficulty reducing fat intake in their diet.

- **Liraglutide (Saxenda):**

  Liraglutide is an injectable medication that mimics a hormone called **GLP-1**, which helps regulate blood sugar and appetite. It can promote weight loss by **reducing hunger** and increasing **satiety** after meals.

- **Naltrexone-Bupropion (Contrave):**

  This combination drug works by targeting areas of the brain involved in **hunger** and **reward**, helping to reduce food cravings. It is particularly useful for individuals who struggle with emotional eating or food addiction.

- **Phentermine-Topiramate (Qsymia):**

  This combination medication includes phentermine and **topiramate**, an anticonvulsant that also aids in weight loss. It may be considered for individuals who have not achieved sufficient results with phentermine alone.

Before considering any alternative medications, patients should consult their healthcare provider to discuss potential benefits and risks, as well as how these medications fit into their overall treatment plan.

---

5. Surgical and Non-Surgical Weight Loss Procedures

For individuals who are severely obese or who have not been successful with medication and lifestyle changes alone, **bariatric surgery** or **non-surgical weight loss procedures** may be an option. These treatments can provide more significant and long-term weight loss results but should be considered carefully, as they come with their own set of risks and requirements.

- **Bariatric Surgery**:

  Bariatric surgery is typically reserved for individuals with a **BMI of 40 or higher** (or 35 and higher with obesity-related health conditions). The most common types of bariatric surgery include:

  - **Gastric Bypass**: This procedure reduces the size of the stomach and reroutes part of the small intestine to limit food intake and absorption.

  - **Gastric Sleeve (Sleeve Gastrectomy)**: This procedure involves removing a portion of the stomach, resulting in a smaller, sleeve-shaped stomach that restricts food intake.

- Adjustable Gastric Banding (Lap-Band): In this procedure, a band is placed around the upper part of the stomach to create a small pouch, limiting the amount of food that can be eaten at one time.

- **Non-Surgical Procedures**:

  For individuals who prefer less invasive options, **non-surgical weight loss procedures** are available. These include:

  - Endoscopic Sleeve Gastroplasty (ESG): A minimally invasive procedure that uses an endoscope to reduce the size of the stomach without the need for incisions.

○ **Gastric Balloon**: A balloon is placed in the stomach and inflated to take up space, helping patients feel full with smaller portions.

While these procedures can lead to significant weight loss, they require a long-term commitment to **dietary changes, exercise, and medical follow-up** to be successful.

---

6. Mind-Body Practices and Stress Management

Stress can play a significant role in weight gain and hinder weight loss efforts. **Mind-body practices** such as **meditation, yoga,** and **deep breathing exercises** can help reduce stress levels, improve mental clarity, and support emotional well-being during the weight loss process.

- **Meditation and Mindfulness**:

  Mindfulness techniques help patients become more aware of their eating habits, emotional triggers, and body cues. Practices like **mindful eating** encourage individuals to eat slowly, savor their food, and listen to their body's signals of hunger and fullness.

- **Yoga and Tai Chi**:

  These gentle forms of exercise not only promote physical activity but also help reduce stress and improve flexibility and balance. Incorporating yoga or tai chi into a weekly routine can enhance **mental and physical well-being,** which supports weight loss goals.

- **Stress Management**:

  Chronic stress can lead to **emotional eating** and weight gain, as the body releases the hormone **cortisol** in response to stress. Finding healthy ways to manage stress, such as through **hobbies, social support**, or **therapy**, is essential for maintaining long-term weight loss.

Conclusion

Incorporating complementary therapies and alternative treatments can significantly enhance the results achieved with Acxion Phentermine. By combining **behavioral therapy, nutritional counseling, physical therapy**, and **mind-body practices**, patients can develop a well-rounded approach to weight management that supports both their physical and emotional health. Exploring **alternative medications** or even considering **surgical** and **non-surgical weight loss**

procedures may also be beneficial for certain individuals who need additional support.

In the next chapter, we will explore real-life **success stories** and examples of individuals who have achieved their weight loss goals with the help of Acxion Phentermine and these complementary approaches.

Chapter 8: Success Stories and Real-Life Results

For many individuals, the journey to losing weight can be long, challenging, and filled with obstacles. However, with the help of **Acxion Phentermine** and a dedicated approach to lifestyle changes, numerous people have been able to achieve significant weight loss and improve their overall health. This chapter will share real-life **success stories**, illustrating how others have overcome barriers and reached their goals.

Each story is unique, highlighting different challenges, approaches, and results. These examples provide insight into the diverse experiences people have had with Acxion Phentermine and offer inspiration for those currently embarking on their own weight loss journey.

Success Story #1: Maria – 40 Pounds Lost in 12 Weeks

Maria, a 35-year-old mother of two, had struggled with weight gain since her pregnancies. Despite multiple attempts to lose weight through dieting and exercise, she found it difficult to stay consistent. Maria's **Body Mass Index (BMI)** was 32, placing her in the obese category, and she was beginning to experience **joint pain** and **fatigue**. Her doctor recommended Acxion Phentermine as part of a **structured weight loss program**.

Initial Challenges:

Maria had developed **emotional eating habits**, often turning to food for comfort when she felt stressed or overwhelmed. She also had difficulty finding time to exercise due to her busy schedule as a working mother.

Plan and Approach:

Maria began taking **Acxion 30 mg** daily, along with making small, manageable changes to her diet. She worked with a **nutritionist** who helped her incorporate more **whole foods**, particularly **lean proteins** and **vegetables**, while reducing her intake of processed foods. She also set a goal to exercise **30 minutes a day**, even if that meant doing simple activities like **walking** around her neighborhood or following an online workout.

Results:

Over the course of **12 weeks**, Maria lost **40 pounds**. The combination of Acxion Phentermine and her new eating habits significantly reduced her appetite, allowing her to stick to a **caloric deficit** without feeling deprived. The joint pain she had experienced also diminished as she lost weight, making exercise more enjoyable. Her success inspired her to continue making healthy choices, even after she stopped taking Acxion.

Maria's Advice:

"Taking Acxion helped me break the cycle of emotional eating and gain control over my appetite. It wasn't easy at first, but once I saw the pounds coming off, I felt more motivated to keep going. The key for me was focusing on small changes, one day at a time."

Success Story #2: John – Overcoming a Plateau

John, a 42-year-old office worker, had been struggling with his weight for several years. He had tried multiple diets and lost 20 pounds on his own, but then hit a **plateau** where he could no longer lose additional weight. John was concerned about his risk for **type 2 diabetes**, as his blood sugar levels were in the **pre-diabetic range**, and he had a family history of the condition.

Initial Challenges:

John found it difficult to maintain his diet because of frequent work lunches and social gatherings. Additionally, his sedentary job made it hard to burn enough calories throughout the day.

Plan and Approach:

After consulting with his healthcare provider, John was prescribed **Acxion 15 mg** to help suppress his appetite. He also worked with a **personal trainer** who created a plan for **strength training** and **cardio exercises** that he could incorporate into his daily routine. John began walking during his lunch breaks and reduced his intake of **sugary snacks** and **refined carbohydrates**.

Results:

Within the first **six weeks** of using Acxion Phentermine, John was able to break through his plateau and lost an additional **25 pounds**. His blood sugar levels improved, and he was able to bring his **A1C levels** back to a healthy range. By focusing on **portion control** and consistent physical activity, John continued to lose weight even after discontinuing Acxion.

John's Advice:

"Acxion gave me the push I needed to break my plateau. The medication helped me control my appetite, and once I saw progress, it was easier to stay motivated. My advice is to focus on creating habits you can stick with long-term, even after you stop taking the medication."

Success Story #3: Ana – Losing Weight with PCOS

Ana, a 28-year-old woman, had struggled with her weight since being diagnosed with **polycystic ovary syndrome (PCOS)** in her early twenties. PCOS made it difficult for her to lose weight due to **hormonal imbalances** that led to **insulin resistance** and increased hunger. Ana's doctor recommended Acxion Phentermine to help her manage her weight and reduce the risk of complications from PCOS, such as **type 2 diabetes**.

Initial Challenges:

Ana often felt hungry, even after eating, which made it challenging to follow a reduced-calorie diet. Her **insulin** resistance also contributed to weight gain, making her feel frustrated with previous attempts to lose weight.

Plan and Approach:

Ana began taking **Acxion 30 mg** in combination with a **low-carbohydrate diet** to help control her insulin levels. Her doctor also recommended regular exercise, including **strength training** and **high-intensity interval training (HIIT)** to improve her insulin sensitivity and metabolism.

Results:

In just **three months**, Ana lost **35 pounds**. The appetite-suppressing effects of Acxion Phentermine helped her stick to her low-carb diet, and her insulin levels improved significantly. Ana also noticed improvements in her **energy levels** and **mood**, as regular exercise became part of her routine.

Ana's Advice:

"Living with PCOS can make weight loss feel impossible, but Acxion helped me get control over my hunger. I focused on balancing my hormones with the right diet and exercise, and that made all the difference. Don't give up—find what works for your body."

Success Story #4: David – Losing Weight for Heart Health

At 55 years old, **David** was facing serious health risks due to his weight. He had been diagnosed with **high blood pressure** and **high cholesterol**, and his doctor warned him that he was at risk for a heart attack. Weighing over 280 pounds, David knew he needed to take control of his health to improve his quality of life.

Initial Challenges:

David's main struggle was a **sedentary lifestyle** and a diet high in **processed foods** and **sodium**, which contributed to his high blood pressure. He often felt fatigued and lacked the energy to exercise.

Plan and Approach:

David's doctor prescribed **Acxion 30 mg** to help reduce his appetite, and he began working with a **dietitian** to lower his intake of **salt, processed foods**, and **sugary drinks**. He also started a **walking program**, slowly increasing his activity level each week.

Results:

In the first **three months**, David lost **50 pounds**, and his **blood pressure** and **cholesterol levels** improved dramatically. He continued to lose weight over the next several months, reaching a total weight loss of **70 pounds**. His doctor was able to reduce his blood pressure medication, and David reported feeling more energized and motivated to continue exercising.

David's Advice:

"For me, it wasn't just about losing weight—it was about getting healthy for my family. Acxion helped me control my cravings, and once I started seeing results, I had the energy to stick with my new lifestyle. If you're struggling, take it one step at a time and remember why you started."

Lessons from Success Stories

These success stories demonstrate the diverse ways in which Acxion Phentermine can be used as part of a comprehensive weight loss plan. While each individual faced different challenges, there are common themes that contributed to their success:

1. **Commitment to Lifestyle Changes**:

   Each person made significant changes to their diet and physical activity levels, recognizing that Acxion Phentermine is most effective when paired with a healthy lifestyle.

2. **Personalized Plans**:

   Working with healthcare professionals such as **nutritionists**, **trainers**, and **therapists** helped these individuals create plans that were tailored to their unique needs and health conditions.

3. **Consistency and Persistence**:

   Weight loss is a gradual process, and all of the individuals highlighted in these stories showed persistence, staying committed to their goals even when faced with challenges.

4. **Long-Term Focus:**

While Acxion Phentermine provided an initial boost, the key to lasting success was adopting sustainable habits that could be maintained after the medication was discontinued.

Conclusion

The success stories shared in this chapter illustrate the transformative impact that Acxion Phentermine can have when used as part of a comprehensive weight loss program. By combining medication with healthy eating, exercise, and ongoing support, individuals can achieve their weight loss goals and improve their overall health.

In the final chapter, we will discuss whether **Acxion Phentermine** is the right option for you and provide guidance on how to work with your healthcare provider to develop a personalized weight loss plan.

Chapter 9: Is Acxion Phentermine Right for You?

As we have explored throughout this book, **Acxion Phentermine** can be an effective tool for weight loss when used under proper medical supervision and combined with healthy lifestyle changes. However, the decision to use Acxion Phentermine should be made carefully, taking into account your individual health status, weight loss goals, and willingness to make long-term changes.

In this final chapter, we will summarize the key considerations that can help you determine whether Acxion Phentermine is right for you and how to move forward with a comprehensive weight management plan.

---

1. Assessing Your Weight Loss Goals

Before considering Acxion Phentermine, it's essential to have a clear understanding of your **weight loss goals**. Are you looking to lose a significant amount of weight due to **health concerns**, such as diabetes or hypertension, or are you seeking to make moderate weight changes for overall wellness? Setting **realistic, measurable, and time-bound goals** will help you decide whether this medication fits into your plan.

- **Who Might Benefit from Acxion Phentermine?**

    Acxion Phentermine is most commonly prescribed for individuals with a **Body Mass Index (BMI) of 30 or higher**, or those with a **BMI of 27 or higher** who also have weight-related health conditions, such as **high blood pressure, type 2 diabetes**, or **sleep apnea**. If your weight is affecting your health or quality of life,

Acxion Phentermine may be an option worth discussing with your healthcare provider.

- **What Are Your Long-Term Objectives?**

Acxion Phentermine is intended for **short-term use**, typically up to **12 weeks**, so it's important to consider how you will maintain weight loss once you stop taking the medication. Developing sustainable habits that focus on **healthy eating, regular physical activity**, and **behavioral changes** will be key to your long-term success.

---

2. Are You Ready for Lifestyle Changes?

As emphasized throughout this book, Acxion Phentermine is not a standalone solution for weight loss. It is most effective when used as part of a broader **lifestyle modification** plan. Ask yourself the following questions to determine if you are ready for the commitment:

- **Are You Prepared to Change Your Diet?**

  Successful weight loss requires not just reducing calories but also improving the **quality of the foods you eat.** Are you willing to adopt a diet rich in **lean proteins, whole grains, fruits,** and **vegetables,** while limiting **processed foods** and **sugary snacks?**

- **Can You Commit to Regular Exercise?**

  Physical activity is essential for losing weight and maintaining long-term results. Are you able to set aside time for **daily exercise,** whether it's walking, strength training, or engaging in an activity you enjoy? Starting with small, manageable changes and gradually increasing intensity can help you build an exercise routine that works for your lifestyle.

- **Are You Open to Behavioral Support?**

  For many individuals, weight loss involves addressing **emotional eating, stress,** and other psychological factors. Would you be willing to explore **behavioral therapy, counseling,** or **support groups** to help you overcome these challenges? Building a support system, whether through professionals or peers, can provide accountability and motivation during your journey.

---

3. Understanding the Risks and Benefits

Acxion Phentermine, like all medications, comes with potential **risks** and **side effects,** which have been discussed in earlier chapters. Before deciding to use this medication, it's crucial to weigh the benefits against the risks, particularly if you have underlying health conditions.

- **Potential Benefits**:
  - Helps **suppress appetite**, making it easier to stick to a low-calorie diet.
  - Provides a **kick-start** to weight loss, which can be motivating.
  - Can improve health conditions related to obesity, such as **high blood pressure, high cholesterol,** and **insulin resistance**.

- **Potential Risks**:
  - Side effects like **dry mouth, insomnia, increased heart rate,** and **elevated blood pressure**.

○ Risk of **dependency** with prolonged use, as Acxion Phentermine is a **Schedule IV controlled substance.**

○ Not suitable for individuals with certain medical conditions, such as **heart disease, uncontrolled hypertension, glaucoma,** or **pregnancy.**

Working closely with your healthcare provider will help you evaluate these risks and determine whether Acxion Phentermine is a safe and appropriate option for you.

---

4. Finding the Right Support System

Weight loss is not just about taking medication; it's about creating a supportive environment that encourages lasting change. Your healthcare provider can help you design a

personalized weight loss plan, but having the right support system at home and in your community is equally important.

- **Work with Professionals**:

  Collaborating with a **registered dietitian**, **personal trainer**, or **therapist** can provide guidance and accountability. These professionals can help you navigate challenges and offer expert advice tailored to your needs.

- **Join a Support Group**:

  Connecting with others who are also working towards weight loss can be highly motivating. Whether through **online forums, in-person support groups**, or **social media**, having a community to share experiences, tips, and encouragement can help you stay focused and committed.

- **Enlist the Help of Family and Friends**:

  Involving your loved ones in your weight loss journey can make a big difference. Whether it's through **meal planning, exercising together,** or simply offering emotional support, having people who understand and encourage your efforts will help keep you on track.

---

5. The Role of Medical Supervision

Acxion Phentermine is a prescription medication that requires **close medical supervision** to ensure safe and effective use. It's important to work with a healthcare provider who understands your medical history and can monitor your progress throughout the course of treatment.

- **Initial Assessment**:

  Before starting Acxion Phentermine, your doctor will conduct a thorough **medical evaluation** to determine whether the medication is appropriate for you. This may include reviewing your **BMI, blood pressure, blood sugar levels**, and any existing health conditions.

- **Ongoing Monitoring**:

  During treatment, regular check-ups are essential to monitor **weight loss progress**, manage any side effects, and adjust the dosage if necessary. Your doctor will also check for any signs of **increased blood pressure** or **heart rate** to ensure your safety.

- **Post-Treatment Follow-Up**:

  Once you stop taking Acxion Phentermine, it's important to continue seeing your healthcare provider to

maintain weight loss and prevent regain. They can help you transition to a long-term weight maintenance plan, provide support, and address any concerns that arise after discontinuation of the medication.

---

6. Moving Forward: Is Acxion Phentermine Right for You?

The decision to use Acxion Phentermine is highly personal and should be based on a combination of factors, including your current health, weight loss goals, and ability to make lasting lifestyle changes. For many individuals, Acxion Phentermine can provide the **initial push** needed to break through barriers and start seeing progress. However, it is important to remember that the medication is just one part of the equation.

Consider the following as you make your decision:

- **Are you motivated to make lasting lifestyle changes, including diet and exercise?**

- **Do you understand the risks and benefits of Acxion Phentermine and feel comfortable using the medication under medical supervision?**

- **Are you prepared to work with a healthcare provider and other professionals to develop a comprehensive, sustainable weight loss plan?**

If the answer is yes, Acxion Phentermine could be an effective tool to help you reach your weight loss goals. If you are still unsure, consult your healthcare provider to discuss your concerns and explore alternative options that may be better suited to your needs.

Conclusion: Sustaining Weight Loss Long-Term

Regardless of whether you choose to use Acxion Phentermine or pursue other weight loss methods, the ultimate goal is to develop habits that will help you achieve and maintain a healthy weight over the long term. Success in weight loss is about **consistency**, **commitment**, and a willingness to make gradual changes that will benefit your health in the years to come.

- **Focus on Sustainable Habits**:

  Quick fixes rarely lead to lasting results. Instead, prioritize **small, sustainable changes** that you can maintain over time. These might include cooking more meals at home, walking daily, or practicing mindful eating.

- **Track Your Progress**:

  Keeping track of your food intake, exercise, and weight loss can help you stay accountable and motivated. It also allows you to identify areas where you may need to make adjustments.

- **Stay Flexible and Adapt**:

  Weight loss journeys are rarely linear, and you may encounter setbacks along the way. Be patient with yourself and stay open to adapting your plan as needed. Remember, the goal is to create a healthy, balanced lifestyle that you can enjoy and sustain.

- **Celebrate Your Wins**:

  Whether it's reaching a weight loss milestone, improving your blood pressure, or simply feeling more energized, take time to celebrate your achievements. Recognizing your progress, no matter how small, will keep you motivated to continue.

Final Thoughts

Acxion Phentermine can be a powerful tool for initiating weight loss, but its true effectiveness comes from combining it with a comprehensive approach that includes **dietary changes, exercise**, and **behavioral support**. If you are ready to take the next step in your weight loss journey, start by talking to your healthcare provider to see if Acxion Phentermine is the right option for you.

Remember, the journey to better health is not a sprint—it's a marathon. Stay committed, stay patient, and trust in the process. With the right mindset and support, you can achieve

your weight loss goals and enjoy a healthier, more fulfilling life.

Made in the USA
Las Vegas, NV
11 November 2024